Eyesight Improvement

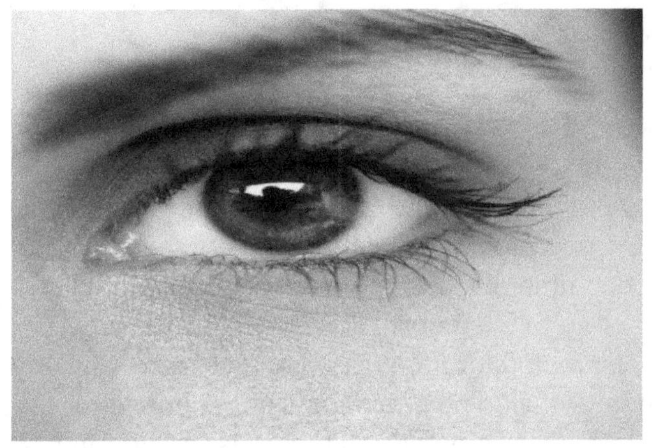

A Comprehensive Guide to Eye
Health and Good Vision with Vitamins
and Supplements

Isaac Hendricks

Table of Contents

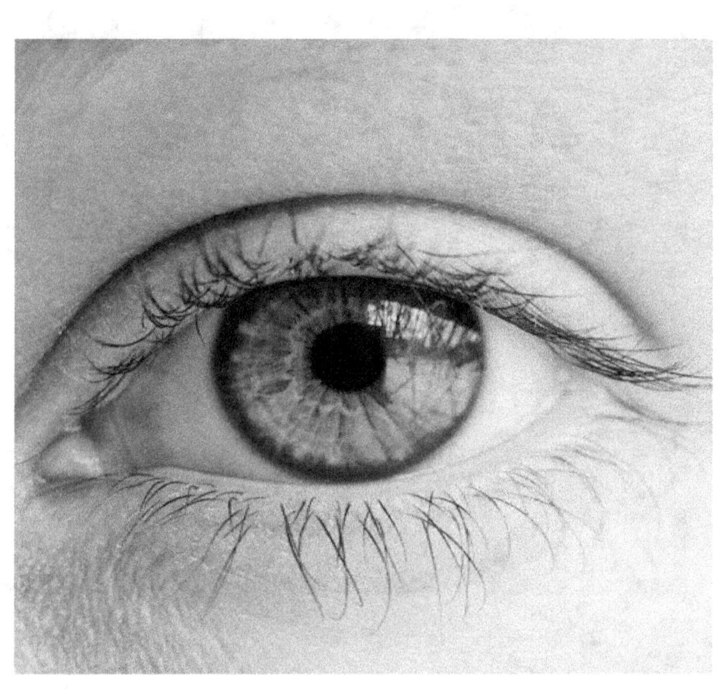

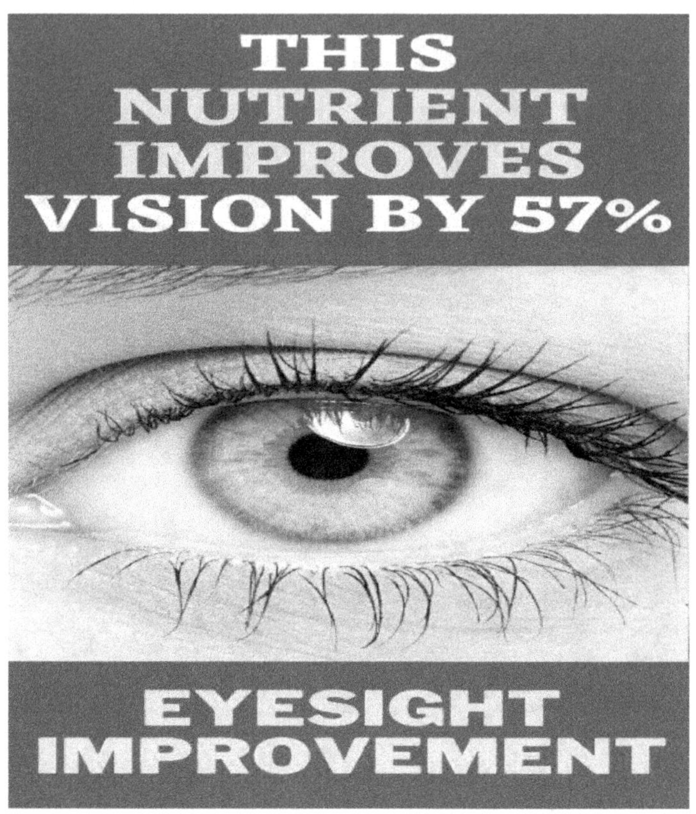
THIS
NUTRIENT
IMPROVES
VISION BY 57%
EYESIGHT
IMPROVEMENT

INTRODUCTION

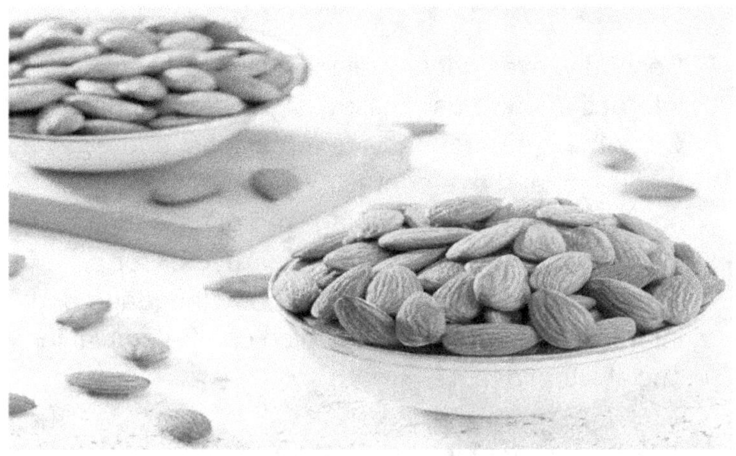

Importance of Eyesight

Eyesight is one of the most valuable senses that humans possess. It allows us to perceive the world around us, navigate through our surroundings, and interact with others. Without eyesight, our lives would be vastly different and much more challenging. In this essay, I will discuss the importance of eyesight and why it is crucial for our daily lives.

Firstly, eyesight is essential for our survival. It helps us to avoid danger and navigate through unfamiliar environments. For instance, when we are walking in a new place, our eyesight enables us to spot potential hazards like potholes, obstacles, or pedestrians crossing the road. This ability to see and react quickly is crucial for our safety and well-being.

Secondly, eyesight is vital for our social interactions. We use our eyesight to communicate with others through facial expressions, body language, and eye contact. When we meet someone new, the first thing we notice is their appearance, which includes their eyes. Our eyesight also helps us to read body language and interpret non-verbal cues, which can be crucial in social situations.

Thirdly, eyesight is essential for learning and education. It allows us to read books, study textbooks, and watch educational videos. Without eyesight, learning would be much more challenging as we would not be able to read or see visual aids like diagrams or charts. This would hinder our academic progress and limit our opportunities for personal growth and development.

Fourthly, eyesight is crucial for our professional lives. It helps us to perform tasks accurately and efficiently in various professions like medicine, engineering, and design. For example, doctors use their eyesight to diagnose diseases and injuries by examining medical images like X-rays or MRI scans. Engineers use their eyesight to design complex structures and machines by visualising them in three dimensions. Designers use their eyesight to create visually appealing products by selecting colours, shapes, and textures that complement each other.

Lastly, eyesight is essential for our overall health and well-being. It helps us to maintain a healthy lifestyle by enabling us to make informed decisions about our diet, exercise routine, and medical care. For instance, we can see if we are eating enough fruits and vegetables by looking at their colours and textures. We can also see if we are getting enough exercise by monitoring our heart rate or breathing patterns during physical activity. Moreover, we can detect early signs of diseases like cataracts or glaucoma by regularly getting an eye check-up from an ophthalmologist.

In conclusion, eyesight is a crucial sense that plays a significant role in our daily lives. It helps us to survive, communicate, learn, work, and maintain good health. Therefore, it is essential to take care of our eyesight by eating a healthy diet rich in vitamins A and C, protecting them from UV rays by wearing sunglasses or hats with brims, quitting smoking or avoiding secondhand smoke exposure, getting regular eye check-ups from an ophthalmologist every two years (or annually if you have a family history of eye diseases), and practising good hygiene habits like washing your hands frequently to prevent the spread of eye infections like conjunctivitis (pink eye). By taking these simple steps, we can preserve our eyesight for a lifetime and enjoy the beauty of the world around us.

Common Eye Problems

Eyes are one of the most important senses that allow us to perceive the world around us. However, just like any other body part, eyes can also develop various problems that can affect our vision and overall eye health. In this article, we will discuss some common eye problems that people may experience.

1. Myopia (Near-Sightedness)

Myopia, also known as near-sightedness, is a common eye problem that affects millions of people worldwide. In this condition, the person can see nearby objects clearly but has difficulty seeing distant objects. This happens because the light entering the eye focuses in front of the retina instead of on it, causing blurred vision. Myopia is often caused by genetics and lifestyle factors such as excessive screen time and reading in low light conditions.

2. Hyperopia (Far-Sightedness)

Hyperopia, also known as far-sightedness, is another common eye problem that affects people's vision. In this condition, the person can see distant objects clearly but has difficulty seeing nearby objects. This happens because the light entering the eye focuses behind the retina instead of on it, causing blurred vision. Hyperopia is often caused by genetics and lifestyle factors such as excessive screen time and reading in low light conditions.

3. Astigmatism

Astigmatism is a condition where the curvature of the cornea or lens is irregular, causing blurred vision at all distances. This condition can occur in combination with myopia or hyperopia or on its own. Astigmatism can be caused by genetics or other factors such as eye injuries or surgery.

4. Presbyopia

Presbyopia is an age-related eye problem that affects people's ability to focus on nearby objects. This condition occurs when the lens inside the eye loses its flexibility, making it difficult to focus on close objects. Presbyopia usually starts to develop in people in their mid-forties and can be corrected with reading glasses or contact lenses.

5. Cataracts

Cataracts are a common eye problem that affects the lens inside the eye, causing it to become cloudy and opaque over time. This condition can lead to blurred vision and eventually complete blindness if left untreated. Cataracts are often caused by ageing, but they can also be caused by other factors such as diabetes, smoking, and UV radiation exposure.

6. Glaucoma

Glaucoma is a serious eye condition that affects the optic nerve, causing damage to the nerve fibres that transmit visual information from the eye to the brain. This condition can lead to permanent vision loss if left untreated. Glaucoma is often caused by high intraocular pressure (IOP), but it can also be caused by other factors such as ageing and family history of glaucoma.

7. Dry Eye Syndrome

Dry Eye Syndrome is a common eye problem that affects people's tear production and quality, causing dryness, irritation, and discomfort in the eyes. This condition can be caused by various factors such as ageing, medications, and environmental factors such as dry air or windy conditions.

In conclusion, these are some common eye problems that people may experience at different stages of their lives. It's essential to maintain good eye health by getting regular eye exams, protecting your eyes from UV radiation exposure, quitting smoking, eating a healthy diet rich in vitamins A and C, and practising good hygiene habits such as washing your hands frequently to prevent eye infections. If you experience any symptoms of these conditions or have concerns about your eye health, it's best to consult with an ophthalmologist for proper diagnosis and treatment options.

Benefits of Improving Eyesight

Improving eyesight is not just about being able to see clearly without the aid of glasses or contact lenses. It has numerous benefits that go beyond just visual acuity. Here are some of the advantages of enhancing eyesight:

1. Reduced Risk of Eye Diseases: When you improve your eyesight, you reduce the risk of developing eye diseases such as cataracts, glaucoma, and macular degeneration. These conditions are often associated with ageing, but they can be prevented or delayed by maintaining good eye health through regular eye exams, a healthy diet, and lifestyle changes.

2. Improved Overall Health:
The eyes are a window to the body's overall health. Many systemic diseases such as diabetes, high blood pressure, and high cholesterol can be detected through eye exams. By improving your eyesight, you may also be able to detect these diseases earlier and take appropriate action to manage them.

3. Enhanced Learning and Cognitive Function:
The eyes play a crucial role in learning and cognitive function. Children with poor vision may have difficulty learning and may fall behind in school. Adults with poor vision may have trouble reading, working on computers, or driving, which

can impact their productivity and quality of life. By improving eyesight, you can enhance learning and cognitive function, making it easier to learn new skills and perform daily tasks.

4. Increased Safety:

Poor vision can pose a significant safety risk in various situations such as driving, crossing the street, or working with machinery. By improving eyesight, you can reduce the risk of accidents and injuries caused by poor vision.

5. Improved Quality of Life:

Good vision is essential for enjoying life's pleasures such as reading a book, watching a movie, or playing sports. By improving eyesight, you can enjoy these activities without the aid of glasses or contact lenses, making it more convenient and cost-effective in the long run.

In conclusion, improving eyesight has numerous benefits beyond just visual acuity. It reduces the risk of eye diseases, improves overall health, enhances learning and cognitive function, increases safety, and improves the quality of life. By taking steps to maintain good eye health through regular eye exams, a healthy diet, and lifestyle changes, you can enjoy these benefits and lead a healthier and happier life.

CHAPTER ONE

Natural Ways to Improve Eyesight

Exercises for Eyesight Improvement

As we spend more time staring at screens and digital devices, our eyesight is increasingly becoming a concern. The constant strain on our eyes can lead to eye fatigue, headaches, and even vision problems like myopia (nearsightedness) and astigmatism. Fortunately, there are several exercises that can help improve eyesight naturally. Here are a few of the most effective:

1. Palming: This exercise involves closing your eyes and placing your palms over your eyelids. Take deep breaths and relax your body as you do this. This exercise helps to reduce eye strain and fatigue by promoting relaxation and improving blood flow to the eyes.

2. Blinking: Blinking is an essential part of maintaining healthy eyesight, but many people blink less frequently when using digital devices. Try blinking more often, especially when working on a screen for long periods. This exercise helps to lubricate the eyes and prevent dryness and irritation.

3. Eye Rotations: Sit comfortably with your eyes closed, then slowly rotate your eyes clockwise in a circular motion for 10 seconds. Repeat the exercise in an anticlockwise direction for another 10 seconds. This exercise helps to improve eye coordination and reduce eye fatigue.

4. Focusing Exercises: Hold an object at arm's length, then focus on it for 10 seconds. Move the object closer to your face until it's about 10 inches away, then focus on it for another 10 seconds. Repeat this exercise several times a day to improve focusing ability.

5. Near-Far Exercises: Hold a pen or pencil at arm's length, then focus on it for 10 seconds. Move the object closer to your face until it's about 10 inches away, then focus on it for another 10 seconds. Move the object further away from your face until it's about an arm's length away, then focus on it for another 10 seconds. Repeat this exercise several times a day to improve near-far focusing ability.

6. Sunning: Sit in a sunny spot with your eyes closed, then open them slowly as you look up at the sky. Focus on the brightness of the sun or sky for about 30 seconds, then close your eyes again and repeat the exercise several times a day. This exercise helps to improve eye health by increasing blood flow and oxygenation to the eyes.

7. Reading: Reading is an excellent way to improve eyesight as it involves focusing on small print for extended periods. Try reading a book or magazine without glasses or contacts if you wear them, as this can help strengthen your vision over time.

Incorporating these exercises into your daily routine can help improve eyesight naturally without relying on corrective lenses or surgery. Remember to take breaks from screens frequently and practise good posture when working or studying to further promote healthy eyesight habits!

Foods for Better Eyesight

Maintaining good eyesight is crucial for our daily activities, and a healthy diet plays a significant role in promoting eye health. Several foods are rich in nutrients that can improve eyesight and prevent age-related eye diseases such as cataracts and macular degeneration. Here are some of the best foods for better eyesight:

- Leafy Greens: Leafy greens such as spinach, kale, and collard greens are packed with vitamin A, which is essential for healthy eyes. Vitamin A helps to produce rhodopsin, a protein that enables us to see in low light conditions.

- Carrots: Carrots are rich in beta-carotene, a precursor to vitamin A. Beta-carotene helps to protect the eyes from oxidative damage and reduces the risk of cataracts and macular degeneration.

- Berries: Berries such as blueberries, strawberries, and raspberries contain antioxidants called anthocyanins, which protect the eyes from UV radiation and reduce inflammation.

- Nuts and Seeds: Nuts and seeds such as almonds, walnuts, chia seeds, and flaxseeds are rich in omega-3 fatty acids, which are essential for maintaining healthy eyes. Omega-3s help to reduce inflammation and prevent dry eyes.

- Fatty Fish: Fatty fish such as salmon, mackerel, and sardines are rich in omega-3 fatty acids and vitamin D, both of which are essential for eye health. Vitamin D helps to prevent cataracts and macular degeneration.

- Eggs: Eggs are rich in lutein and zeaxanthin, two antioxidants that help to protect the eyes from UV radiation and reduce the risk of cataracts and macular degeneration.

- Sweet Potatoes: Sweet potatoes are rich in beta-carotene, which is converted into vitamin A in the body. Vitamin A helps to prevent night blindness and reduces the risk of cataracts.

- Citrus Fruits: Citrus fruits such as oranges, lemons, and grapefruits are rich in vitamin C, which helps to prevent cataracts and macular degeneration by reducing oxidative stress.

Incorporating these foods into your diet can significantly improve your eyesight and promote overall eye health. Remember to eat a balanced diet that includes a variety of fruits, vegetables, whole grains, lean proteins, and healthy fats to maintain optimal eye health.

Herbal Remedies for Eyesight Improvement

Herbal remedies have been used for centuries to improve eyesight and promote overall eye health. While modern medicine offers various treatments for vision problems, many people prefer natural remedies due to their perceived safety and potential benefits. In this article, we will explore some of the most popular herbal remedies for eyesight improvement.

Bilberry (Vaccinium myrtillus)

Bilberry is a type of blueberry that is native to Europe. It contains anthocyanins, which are antioxidant compounds that help protect the eyes from damage caused by free radicals. Studies have shown that bilberry extract can improve night vision and reduce eye fatigue. It is also believed to help prevent cataracts and macular degeneration.

Ginkgo biloba

Ginkgo biloba is a Chinese tree that has been utilised in traditional Chinese medicine for thousands of years. It contains flavonoids and terpenoids, which are antioxidant compounds that help protect the eyes from damage caused by free radicals. Studies have shown that ginkgo biloba extract can improve visual acuity and reduce symptoms of age-related macular degeneration.

Turmeric (Curcuma longa)

Turmeric is a spice that is often used in Indian cooking. It contains curcumin, which is a powerful antioxidant compound that helps protect the eyes from damage caused by free radicals. Studies have shown that curcumin can improve visual acuity and reduce symptoms of age-related macular degeneration.

Spirulina (Arthrospira platensis)

Spirulina is a type of blue-green algae that is rich in nutrients such as beta-carotene, vitamin A, and antioxidants. Studies have shown that spirulina can improve visual acuity and reduce symptoms of cataracts.

Eyebright (Euphrasia officinalis)
Eyebright is a herb commonly used in traditional medicine to treat eye problems such as conjunctivitis and blepharitis. It contains flavonoids and tannins, which help reduce inflammation and promote healing of the eyes. Studies have shown that eyebright extract can improve visual acuity and reduce symptoms of dry eye syndrome.

Rosehip (Rosa canina)
Rosehip is the fruit of the rose plant that is rich in vitamin A, vitamin C, and antioxidants. Studies have shown that rosehip extract can improve visual acuity and reduce symptoms of cataracts.

Acai berry (Euterpe oleracea)
Acai berry is a fruit commonly found in the rainforest that is rich in antioxidants such as anthocyanins and flavonoids. Studies have shown that acai berry extract can improve visual acuity and reduce symptoms of age-related macular degeneration.

It's important to note that while herbal remedies may offer potential benefits for eyesight improvement, they should not replace medical treatment for serious eye conditions such as cataracts or glaucoma. It's always best to consult with a healthcare professional before trying any new herbal remedies, especially if you have underlying health conditions or are taking prescription medications.

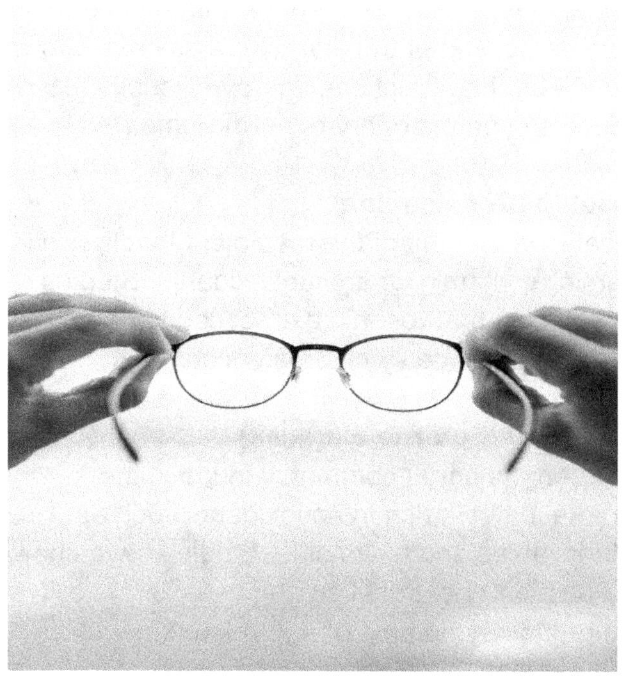

CHAPTER TWO

Eye Care Tips

Protecting Your Eyes from UV Rays

In today's world, where technology and screens have become an integral part of our daily lives, it's essential to take care of our eyes. One of the most significant threats to our eye health is ultraviolet (UV) radiation. UV rays are a type of electromagnetic radiation that comes from the sun and other artificial sources like tanning beds and fluorescent lights. Prolonged exposure to UV radiation can lead to various eye problems, including cataracts, macular degeneration, and photokeratitis (sunburn of the eye). In this article, we will discuss some ways to protect your eyes from UV rays.

- Wear Sunglasses:

The most efficient technique to protect your eyes from UV rays is to wear sunglasses. Look for sunglasses that block 99-100% of both UVA and UVB radiation. Wraparound sunglasses are ideal as they protect your eyes from the side as well.

- Wear a Hat:

Wearing a hat with a brim can provide additional protection for your eyes by blocking the sun's rays from above and from the side. This is especially important if you spend a lot of time outdoors or in areas with high UV index.

- Stay Indoors During Peak Hours:

The sun's beams are at their brightest between 10 a.m. and 4 p.m. If possible, avoid being outside during these hours, particularly in areas with high UV index. If you must be outside during these hours, wear sunglasses and a hat for added protection.

- Use UV-Blocking Contact Lenses:

If you wear contact lenses, consider using lenses that offer UV protection. These lenses can help protect your eyes from UV rays and reduce the risk of eye damage.

- Protect Your Eyes During Winter:

Many people believe that UV rays are not a concern during winter because the sun is not as strong. However, snow reflects up to 80% of UV radiation, which can increase your exposure to UV rays during winter months. Therefore, it's essential to wear sunglasses and a hat during winter as well.

- Get Regular Eye Exams:

Regular eye exams are necessary for maintaining good eye health. During an eye exam, your optometrist can check for signs of eye damage caused by UV radiation and recommend appropriate measures to protect your eyes.

In conclusion, protecting your eyes from UV rays is crucial for maintaining good eye health. By following the tips mentioned above, you can significantly reduce your risk of developing eye problems caused by UV radiation. Remember to wear sunglasses, a hat, stay indoors during peak hours, use UV-blocking contact lenses, protect your eyes during winter, and get regular eye exams. Your eyes will thank you!

Maintaining a Healthy Lifestyle

Maintaining a healthy lifestyle is crucial for overall well-being, and it's particularly important for preserving and improving eyesight. Our eyes are delicate organs that require special care and attention in order to work properly. Here are some tips for maintaining a healthy lifestyle for eyesight improvement:

1. Eat a balanced diet: A healthy diet rich in vitamins and minerals is essential for maintaining good eyesight. Foods that are particularly beneficial for eye health include leafy green vegetables, citrus fruits, nuts, and fatty fish like salmon. These foods contain antioxidants, vitamins A, C, and E, and omega-3 fatty acids, which help protect the eyes from damage and improve vision.

2. Exercise regularly: Regular exercise can help improve blood flow to the eyes, which is essential for maintaining good eyesight. Exercise also helps reduce stress, which can contribute to eye strain and fatigue.

3. Get enough sleep: Getting enough sleep is crucial for maintaining good eyesight. During sleep, the body repairs itself, including the eyes. Lack of sleep can lead to eye strain, fatigue, and dryness, which can negatively impact vision.

4. Protect your eyes from UV rays: Exposure to UV rays can damage the eyes and contribute to age-related macular degeneration (AMD), a condition that can lead to vision loss. Wear sunglasses with UV protection when outdoors, especially during peak UV hours (10 am to 4 pm).

5. Quit smoking: Smoking is a major risk factor for eye diseases like cataracts and AMD. Quitting smoking can significantly reduce the risk of developing these conditions and improve overall eye health.

6. Manage chronic conditions: Chronic conditions like diabetes and high blood pressure can negatively impact eye health and contribute to vision loss. Managing these conditions through diet, exercise, and medication can help preserve good eyesight.

7. Get regular eye exams: Regular eye exams are essential for maintaining good eyesight and detecting any underlying eye conditions early on. Schedule an eye exam with an optometrist or ophthalmologist at least once a year, especially if you have a family history of eye diseases or are over the age of 60.

By following these tips, you can maintain a healthy lifestyle that promotes good eyesight and reduces the risk of developing eye diseases later in life. Remember to prioritise your eye health as part of your overall wellness routine!

Tips for Computer Users to Prevent Eye Strain

As technology has advanced, the use of computers and digital devices has become an integral part of our daily lives. However, prolonged use of these devices can lead to eye strain, headaches, and other vision problems. Here are some tips for computer users to prevent eye strain:

Adjust the brightness and contrast

Make sure your computer screen's brightness and contrast are adjusted to match the lighting in your workspace. This will assist in reducing eye strain and fatigue.

Blink more

Blinking helps keep your eyes moisturised and prevents dryness, which can lead to eye strain. Make a conscious effort to blink more frequently while using your computer.

Take breaks

It's essential to take regular breaks from your computer screen. The 20-20-20 rule is a popular method for preventing eye strain. Look away from your screen for 20 seconds every 20 minutes and at an object 20 feet away.

Adjust the font size

Make sure the font size on your computer is large enough to read comfortably without straining your eyes. You can also adjust the text color and background colour to make it easier on your eyes.

Use anti-glare screens

Anti-glare screens can significantly reduce glare and reflections, making it easier on your eyes when working in bright environments.

Position your screen correctly

Your computer screen should be positioned directly in front of you, about an arm's length away, and slightly below eye level. This will reduce neck and eye strain.

Use proper lighting

Make sure your workspace is well-lit, but avoid direct light sources that can create glare on your screen.

Get regular eye exams

Regular eye exams are essential to maintain good eye health and catch any vision problems early on. If you experience any vision problems while using your computer, consult with an eye care professional for advice on how to manage them.

By following these tips, you can significantly reduce the risk of eye strain and other vision problems associated with prolonged computer use. Remember to prioritise taking breaks and practising good posture while using your computer to prevent neck and back strain as well!

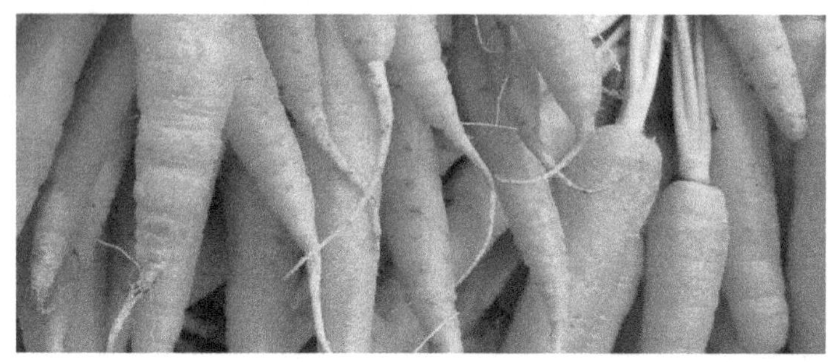

VITAMINS
For Your Eyes

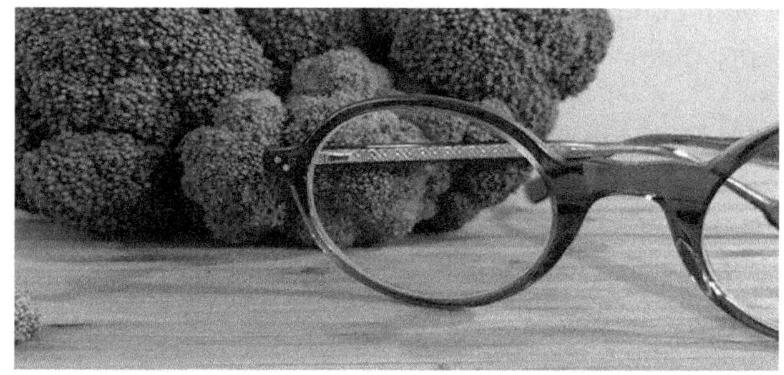

CHAPTER THREE

Corrective Measures for Common Eye Problems

Myopia (Nearsightedness)

Myopia, often known as nearsightedness, is a vision disorder that affects millions of people around the world. It occurs when the eye's shape prevents light from focusing precisely on the retina, causing distant objects to appear blurry while nearby objects remain clear. The exact cause of myopia is not fully understood, but several factors are believed to contribute to its development.

One of the primary factors that may lead to myopia is genetics. Individuals with a family history of nearsightedness are more likely to develop the problem themselves, according to research. Additionally, environmental factors such as excessive screen time, lack of outdoor activity, and near work may also contribute to myopia's development.

The prevalence of myopia has increased significantly in recent years, particularly in urban areas where people spend more time indoors and less time outdoors. This trend has led some experts to suggest that environmental factors may be playing a more significant role in myopia's development than previously thought.

The impact of myopia on an individual's vision and overall health is significant. In addition to blurry vision at a distance, individuals with myopia are at an increased risk of developing other eye conditions such as cataracts, glaucoma, and retinal detachment. If left untreated, these disorders can result in permanent visual loss.

Fortunately, there are various options for treating and preventing myopia.
One effective method is to encourage children to spend more time outdoors and engage in activities that involve looking at distant objects. This can help strengthen the eye's focusing mechanism and reduce the risk of developing myopia. Additionally, reducing screen time and taking frequent breaks when using digital devices can also help prevent myopia's development.

In cases where myopia has already developed, corrective lenses such as glasses or contact lenses can help improve vision. In some cases, refractive surgery may also be an option for individuals with severe myopia. However, it's essential to consult with an eye care professional to determine the best course of action based on individual needs and circumstances.

In conclusion, myopia is a common vision condition that affects many people worldwide. While genetics may play a role in its development, environmental factors such as excessive screen time and lack of outdoor activity may also contribute. Encouraging children to spend more time outdoors and reducing screen time can help prevent myopia's development. Corrective lenses and refractive surgery are effective methods for managing myopia once it has already developed. It's essential to prioritise regular eye exams and consult with an eye care professional for personalised advice on managing myopia effectively.

Hyperopia (Farsightedness)

Hyperopia, commonly known as farsightedness, is a vision condition where an individual has difficulty focusing on objects that are near. In contrast to myopia (nearsightedness), where nearby objects appear blurry, hyperopia causes distant objects to appear hazy or unfocused. This condition occurs when the eye is too short or the cornea is too flat, causing light to focus behind the retina instead of directly on it.

The symptoms of hyperopia can vary from mild to severe, depending on the degree of the condition. Mild hyperopia may not cause any noticeable symptoms, while severe hyperopia can lead to eye strain, headaches, and fatigue, particularly when reading or working on close tasks for extended periods.

The causes of hyperopia are multifactorial and can be inherited or acquired. Some individuals are born with a shorter than average axial length of the eye, which predisposes them to hyperopia. Others may develop this condition due to ageing or prolonged use of digital devices that cause accommodation fatigue.

Treatment for hyperopia depends on the severity of the condition and the individual's lifestyle needs. In mild cases, no treatment may be necessary, and regular eye exams are recommended to monitor any changes in vision. For moderate to severe hyperopia, corrective lenses such as glasses or contact lenses can help focus light onto the retina accurately. In some cases, surgical interventions such as LASIK or refractive lens exchange may be recommended to correct the condition permanently.

In conclusion, hyperopia (farsightedness) is a common vision condition that affects many individuals worldwide. While mild cases may not require any treatments to severe hyperopia can lead to discomfort and visual impairment. Regular eye exams and appropriate corrective measures can help manage this condition effectively and improve overall visual health.

Presbyopia (Aging-Related Vision Loss)

Presbyopia, also known as age-related farsightedness, is a common vision condition that affects individuals as they age. It typically begins to develop in people around the age of 40 and progresses gradually over time. Presbyopia occurs when the lens of the eye loses its flexibility and ability to focus on nearby objects, making it difficult to read or perform other close-up tasks.

The lens of the eye is responsible for focusing light onto the retina, which is the light-sensitive tissue at the back of the eye. As we age, the lens becomes less elastic and loses its ability to change shape, making it harder for the eye to focus on objects that are close by. This results in blurry vision and requires individuals to hold objects further away in order to see them clearly.

Presbyopia is a natural part of the ageing process and cannot be prevented. However, there are several strategies that can help manage the condition and improve visual function:

1. Eyeglasses or contact lenses: The most common treatment for presbyopia is corrective lenses, which can be worn to help focus light onto the retina. Bifocal or progressive lenses are often prescribed to address both distance and near vision.

2. Reading lights: Bright, focused lighting can help improve visual acuity when reading or performing other close-up tasks.

3. Adjusting workspaces: Placing objects at a comfortable distance and using magnifying glasses can help reduce strain on the eyes and improve clarity.

4. Regular eye exams: It's important to have regular eye exams to monitor changes in vision and ensure that corrective lenses are up-to-date.

Presbyopia is a common condition that affects many individuals as they age, but there are strategies that can help manage the condition and improve visual function. By working with an eye care professional and implementing these strategies, individuals can continue to enjoy clear vision and maintain their quality of life as they grow older.

CHAPTER FOUR

Surgical Procedures for Eye Conditions

Cataract Surgery

Cataract surgery is a common and highly effective procedure that restores vision in individuals who have developed cataracts, a clouding of the natural lens inside the eye. Cataracts typically develop as a result of ageing, but can also be caused by injury, certain medications, or underlying medical conditions such as diabetes.

The clouded lens is removed during cataract surgery and replaced with an artificial lens known as an intraocular lens (IOL). The surgery is normally performed as an outpatient operation, which means that patients can return home the same day.

The surgery itself is relatively quick and painless, taking around 30 minutes to complete. The surgeon will make a small incision in the eye and use ultrasound or laser technology to break up the cataract and remove it. After that, the IOL is placed into the eye through the same incision.

One of the major benefits of cataract surgery is that it can significantly improve vision, particularly in low-light conditions. Patients may also experience improved colour perception and depth of field. Additionally, cataract surgery has a very high success rate, with over 95% of patients reporting improved vision after the procedure.

However, as with any surgical procedure, there are some risks and potential complications associated with cataract surgery. These can include infection, bleeding, inflammation, and retinal detachment. The surgeon will discuss these risks with the patient beforehand to help them make an informed decision about whether the procedure is right for them.

Overall, cataract surgery is a safe and effective way to restore vision in individuals with cataracts. It can greatly improve quality of life by reducing dependence on glasses or contact lenses and allowing patients to enjoy clearer, more vibrant vision. If you are experiencing symptoms of cataracts or have concerns about your vision, it may be worth discussing cataract surgery with your eye care professional to determine if it is right for you.

Laser Eye Surgery (LASIK)

Laser Eye Surgery, commonly known as LASIK (short for Laser-Assisted In Situ Keratomileusis), is a highly advanced medical procedure that has transformed the way people with vision problems see the world. This revolutionary technology uses a laser to reshape the cornea, the clear front part of the eye, to correct nearsightedness, farsightedness, and astigmatism.

The LASIK procedure is typically performed on an outpatient basis and takes only a few minutes per eye. Before the surgery begins, the patient's eyes are numbed with anaesthetic drops, and a device called a lid speculum is used to keep the eyelids open. The surgeon then creates a small flap in the cornea using a laser or a surgical instrument called a microkeratome. This flap is lifted, and the underlying corneal tissue is reshaped using a laser to correct the refractive error. The flap is then carefully replaced and smoothed over the surface of the eye.

The benefits of LASIK surgery are numerous. Firstly, it provides excellent visual outcomes, with most patients achieving 20/20 vision or better after the procedure. Secondly, it eliminates the need for corrective lenses such as glasses or contact lenses, which can be inconvenient and expensive over time. Thirdly, it is a safe and effective procedure, with a high success rate and low risk of complications.

However, like any medical procedure, LASIK surgery does have some risks and potential side effects. These may include dry eyes, halos around lights, glare or starbursts, temporary blurred vision, and discomfort during the healing process. It is essential to discuss these risks with your surgeon before undergoing the procedure to make an informed decision about whether LASIK is right for you.

In conclusion, Laser Eye Surgery (LASIK) is a highly advanced medical procedure that has revolutionised the way people with vision problems see the world. With its excellent visual outcomes, elimination of corrective lenses, and high success rate, it is an attractive option for many individuals seeking to improve their vision. However, it is essential to weigh the risks and potential side effects against the benefits and discuss these with your surgeon before making a decision about whether LASIK is right for you. If you are considering LASIK surgery, it is recommended that you consult with a qualified ophthalmologist to determine if you are a suitable candidate for this procedure.

CHAPTER FIVE

Prevention of Eye Diseases and Disorders

Eye diseases and disorders can significantly impact an individual's vision and quality of life. Fortunately, many of these conditions can be prevented or managed through proper care and lifestyle choices. In this article, we will discuss some tips for preventing common eye diseases and disorders.

1. Protect your eyes from UV radiation

Exposure to ultraviolet (UV) radiation from the sun and other sources can increase the risk of cataracts, macular degeneration, and other eye problems. To protect your eyes, wear sunglasses with UV protection when outdoors, especially during peak UV hours (10 am to 4 pm). If you wear prescription glasses, consider getting lenses with UV protection as well.

2. Quit smoking

Smoking is a significant risk factor for several eye diseases, including cataracts, macular degeneration, and optic nerve damage. Quitting smoking can significantly reduce your risk of developing these conditions and improve your overall health.

3. Maintain a healthy weight and diet

Being overweight or obese increases the risk of developing diabetes, which can lead to diabetic retinopathy, a serious eye disease that can cause blindness. Maintaining a healthy weight through a balanced diet and regular exercise can help prevent diabetes and other related conditions. A diet rich in leafy green vegetables, fruits, and omega-3 fatty acids may also help prevent macular degeneration.

4. Manage chronic conditions

If you have chronic conditions such as diabetes, high blood pressure, or high cholesterol, it's essential to manage them effectively to reduce the risk of eye problems. Work with your healthcare provider to develop a treatment plan that includes regular eye exams and monitoring for any signs of eye disease.

5. Take breaks from screens

Prolonged exposure to digital screens (such as computers, smartphones, and tablets) can cause eye strain, dry eyes, and other vision problems.

Age-Related Macular Degeneration (AMD)

Age-related macular degeneration (AMD) is a progressive eye condition that affects the macula, which is the central part of the retina responsible for sharp, detailed vision. AMD is a leading cause of vision loss in people over the age of 60, affecting approximately 11 million Americans.

Glaucoma Prevention Strategies

Glaucoma is a degenerative eye illness that, if left untreated, can result in irreparable visual loss. While there is no cure for glaucoma, there are several strategies that individuals can adopt to prevent or delay the onset of this condition. Here are some glaucoma prevention strategies:

1. Regular Eye Exams: The most effective way to prevent glaucoma is to get regular eye exams. It is recommended that individuals over the age of 40 should get an eye exam every two years, and those over 65 should get an exam annually. During the exam, the eye doctor will check for signs of glaucoma and other eye diseases.

2. Maintain a Healthy Weight: Being overweight or obese can increase the risk of developing glaucoma. Therefore, maintaining a healthy weight through a balanced diet and regular exercise can help prevent this condition.

3. Protect Your Eyes: Wear sunglasses with UV protection to shield your eyes from the sun's damaging rays. Additionally, wear protective eyewear when participating in sports or other activities that could cause injury to your eyes.

4. Quit Smoking: Smoking increases the risk of developing glaucoma, as well as other eye diseases such as cataracts and macular degeneration. Quitting smoking can reduce the risk of developing these illnesses greatly.

5. Manage Chronic Conditions: Chronic conditions such as diabetes, high blood pressure, and high cholesterol can increase the risk of developing glaucoma. Managing these conditions through medication, diet, and exercise can help prevent or delay the onset of glaucoma.

6. Limit Alcohol Consumption: Excessive alcohol consumption can increase the pressure in your eyes, which can lead to glaucoma. Limiting alcohol consumption to moderate levels (one drink per day for women and two drinks per day for men) can help prevent this condition.

7. Get Enough Sleep: Getting enough sleep (7-8 hours per night) is essential for overall health and can help prevent glaucoma by reducing stress levels and promoting healthy blood pressure levels.

8. Eat a Healthy Diet: Eating a diet rich in fruits, vegetables, and whole grains can help prevent glaucoma by providing essential nutrients such as vitamin C, vitamin E, and lutein that are beneficial for eye health.

In conclusion, preventing glaucoma requires a combination of lifestyle changes and regular eye exams. By adopting these strategies, individuals can significantly reduce their risk of developing this condition and preserve their vision for years to come.

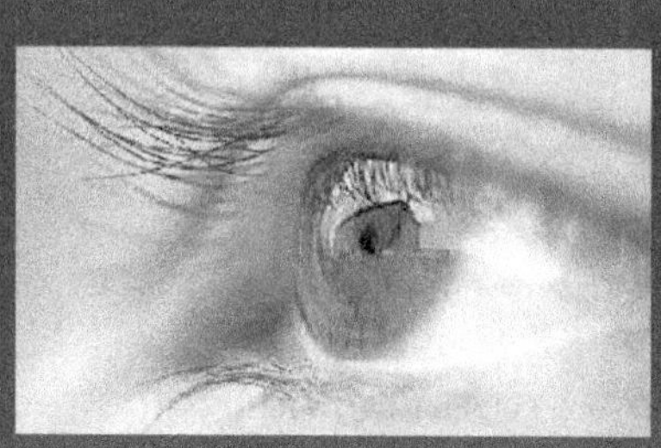

13 food to Improve Eye Vision

1. Carrot
2. Eggs
3. Milk
4. Apricots
5. Berries
6. Black Currants
7. Cold-water Fish
8. Collard Greens
9. Grapefruits
10. Grapes
11. Lemons
12. Spinach
13. Fish Oils

CONCLUSION

In conclusion, the quest for eyesight improvement encompasses a multifaceted approach that spans lifestyle changes, technological interventions, and proactive eye care practices. Through adopting habits like maintaining a balanced diet rich in eye-friendly nutrients, minimising screen time, and incorporating regular eye exercises, individuals can contribute to the preservation and enhancement of their visual acuity. Additionally, advancements in technology, such as blue light filters and vision correction tools, provide valuable tools to alleviate strain and promote ocular health. However, it is crucial to acknowledge the individual variability in responses to these interventions, and consultation with healthcare professionals remains imperative for personalised guidance. As we navigate the digital age, fostering a culture of proactive eye care and embracing a holistic approach to vision health can contribute significantly to the ongoing journey of eyesight improvement.

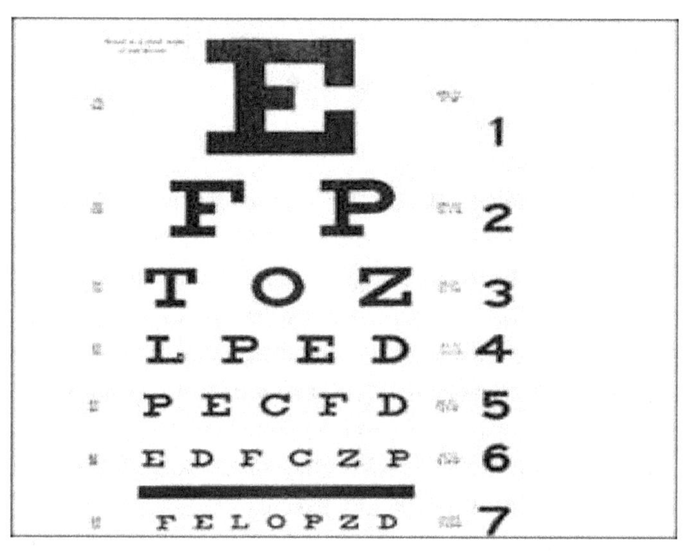

E
F P
T O Z
L P E D
P E C F D
E D F C Z P
F E L O P Z D
1
2
3
4
5
6
7

* 9 7 9 8 8 6 9 9 9 0 9 7 6 *